# THE KETO

## ANTI-INFLAMMATORY

## DIET COOKBOOK

A Comprehensive Guide to Heal Your Body and Reduce Inflammation Through Fat-Fueled, Nutrient-Dense Eating

# Table Of Contents

# Introduction

Chronic inflammation plays a role in almost every major disease from cancer to Alzheimer's. While short-term inflammation is the body's natural response to injury or infection, long-term or chronic inflammation can lead to serious health issues. The good news is that diet and lifestyle changes can help reduce inflammation and its negative impacts.

This book combines the powerful benefits of the ketogenic diet and an anti-inflammatory nutrition plan. The ketogenic or "keto" diet is a low-carb, high-fat way of eating that shifts the body into a metabolic state called ketosis, burning fat rather than glucose for fuel. Keto diets have been shown to reduce inflammation markers in the body.

At the same time, the anti-inflammatory diet focuses on nutrient-dense whole foods like vegetables, fruits, healthy fats, spices, and lean proteins - while limiting foods that promote inflammation such as sugar, refined carbs, unhealthy oils, and processed meats. By following an eating approach that combines keto and anti-inflammatory principles, you can maximize the benefits.

This book will provide you with the essential knowledge about both diets, easy-to-follow meal plans, and delicious recipes that cater to the guidelines of eating keto and anti-inflammatory foods. You'll not only learn how to reduce inflammation through your diet, but also how to achieve all the other benefits of nutritional ketosis such as weight loss, improved energy, better focus and more. Whether you want to reverse an inflammatory condition, achieve better overall health, or simply maximize your body's fat-burning ability, the keto anti-inflammatory approach can get you there. Get ready for a new way of looking at how you eat that can transform your health from the inside out!

# Chapter 1:

# Inspiration

Making the commitment to follow a ketogenic, anti-inflammatory way of eating is one of the most powerful steps you can take to reclaiming your health and vitality. While the journey requires dedication, the potential benefits make it all worthwhile.

Imagine...

Waking up each morning feeling rested and energized rather than groggy and sluggish. Moving through your day with laser-sharp focus and stable energy levels. Having the mental clarity to tackle your biggest goals and dreams.

Picture yourself shedding extra pounds and stubborn weight while simultaneously reducing inflammation that may be impacting chronic conditions or paving the way for future disease. Envision your body operating at its absolute peak.

Think about how rewarding it will feel to prevent cognitive decline and neurodegenerative diseases by nourishing your brain with therapeutic ketones. You're investing in quality of life as you age.

Resolving chronic issues like join pain, skin conditions, digestive problems or autoimmune flare-ups by removing inflammatory dietary triggers could be life-changing. You may finally find relief.

And the best part? All of these transformative benefits stem simply from changing your eating habits to nutrient-dense, whole foods aligned with nutritional ketosis and anti-inflammatory principles. You get to heal your body by enjoying delicious, satisfying meals.

Every forkful of dark leafy greens, succulent fatty fish, or antioxidant-packed berry is an act of self-care. You're making the conscious choice to reduce your risk factors

while optimizing how you look, feel and perform each day. That's incredibly empowering!

So embrace this new lifestyle wholeheartedly. Read the science behind keto and anti-inflammatory nutrition that sparked you to make this change. Follow the meal plans and recipes to make it easily sustainable. And watch in awe as your body begins that healing transformation.

You've got this! Consistency and commitment to nutrient-dense keto living will pay off in ways you've only begun to imagine. Keep that motivating vision top of mind. Your journey towards ultimate health and vitality is finally underway!

# The Benefits of Keto and Anti-Inflammatory Nutrition

By following the principles outlined in this book, you're utilizing two powerful dietary approaches - the ketogenic diet and an anti-inflammatory nutritional plan.

The synergistic combination of these ways of eating can provide a wide range of transformative benefits:

### Reduced Inflammation
At its core, the anti-inflammatory diet removes inflammatory triggers like sugar, refined carbs, unhealthy fats, and processed foods from your meals.

Simultaneously, the keto diet lowers inflammation by regulating blood sugar and eliminating glucose spikes.
This multi-pronged approach is key for managing chronic inflammatory conditions.

### Sustainable Weight Loss
The keto diet has been shown to boost metabolism while providing appetite control through its satiating protein and fat ratios.

It retrains your body to burn fat stores for energy instead of glucose. When combined with the anti-inflammatory whole food focus, this creates an ideal environment for losing weight and keeping it off long-term.

### More Energy and Focus
On keto, your body has a steady supply of

therapeutic ketones for clean-burning fuel.

This provides stable energy without the fatigue and brain fog of glucose/insulin rollercoasters. The anti-inflammatory aspects also support steadier energy by removing disruptive foods.

### Better Gut Health
Both keto and anti-inflammatory diets emphasize fiber-rich vegetables, bone broths, healthy fats like olive oil, and probiotic-rich foods like yogurt. This lineup of gut-friendly foods can favorably impact your microbiome.

### Improved Metabolic Health
This nutritional approach helps reverse insulin resistance, lowering your risk for metabolic issues like type 2 diabetes.
Keto's ability to optimize cholesterol levels is also highly beneficial.

### Reduced Disease Risk
By lowering oxidative stress and regulating inflammatory pathways, you're decreasing your likelihood of developing various chronic diseases from cancer to Alzheimer's to heart disease.

**Better Recovery**

The anti-inflammatory antioxidants coupled with keto's ability to reduce oxidative damage primes your body to recover faster from exercise, injury or surgical procedures.

These are just some of the profound benefits you may experience by embracing the synergy of ketogenic and anti-inflammatory nutrition.

From weight regulation and more energy, to disease prevention and faster recovery - it's an incredibly holistic way to transform your health.

# Keto Diet Food Lists

One of the biggest adjustments when transitioning to a ketogenic diet is changing your grocery shopping habits.

To achieve and remain in a state of nutritional ketosis, you'll need to severely restrict your carb intake while increasing your fat consumption. Here are the key keto-friendly food groups to focus on:

### Fats and Oils
Avocados, avocado oil, olive oil, coconut oil, MCT oil, butter, ghee, lard, tallow, mayonnaise, fatty cuts of meat, fattier fish like salmon.
Proteins
Eggs, beef, lamb, poultry, pork, seafood, jerky, bacon, sausages. Choose fattier cuts where possible.

### Low-Carb Vegetables
Leafy greens, broccoli, cauliflower, zucchini, peppers, mushrooms, tomatoes, onions, garlic, asparagus, eggplant.

### Low-Sugar Fruits
Berries, avocados, olives, lemons, limes in moderation.
Nuts and Seeds
Almonds, walnuts, pecans, chia, flax, pumpkin seeds. Consume in moderation due to carb counts.

### Dairy
Cheese, heavy cream, sour cream, Greek yogurt, butter, ghee.
Drinks

Water, unsweetened seltzers, black coffee, unsweetened teas, bone broth.

### Keto-Friendly Sweeteners
Stevia, monk fruit, erythritol in moderation.
To maintain ketosis, it's recommended to keep net carb intake under 20-30g per day from low-carb veggies, nuts/seeds and small amounts of berries or other low-sugar fruits.

Avoid high-carb foods like grains, legumes, root vegetables, sugar, and sweetened beverages.

With some simple swaps and by focusing on healthy fats, proteins and low-carb plant foods, you can easily build nutrient-dense keto meals and snacks.

# Meal Planning and Preparation Tips

Successful keto and anti-inflammatory eating requires a bit of planning and preparation.

Here are some tips to set yourself up for success:

## Meal Preparation

Taking time once or twice a week to prep keto-friendly foods and meals is a huge timesaver. Grill or bake a batch of chicken, hard-boil eggs, chop veggies, make keto-approved dips and dressings.
Portion into containers for easy grab-and-go options.

## Batch Cooking

Double or triple recipes for protein sources like ground beef, shredded chicken or tuna salad.
Freeze extra portions for quick defrost meals later. Soups, stews and casseroles also make great keto-friendly batch meals.

## Pantry Essentials

Stock your pantry with keto diet staples like olive oil, avocado oil, nut butters, cheese, canned fish, olives, low-carb nuts and seeds, herbs and spices.
This makes meal prep easier.

## Meal Plan

Use the 30-day meal plan in this book or make your own weekly meal plans. This reduces trips to the grocery store and cravings for last-minute takeout. Plan out your meals and snacks.

## Invest in Tools

A good chef's knife, quality pans, air fryer, Instant Pot or slow cooker can all make keto meal prep easier.
Food containers for portioning out meals are also extremely helpful.

## Find Simple Recipes

Focus on easy recipes with fewer ingredients, at least until you get the hang of keto and anti-inflammatory eating patterns.

Simple meat+veggie+healthy fat combos work great.
With a bit of planning each week, you can easily prepare delicious keto-friendly, anti-inflammatory meals that fuel you and reduce inflammation. Meal prepping is key to success!

## Keto Diet Essentials

The ketogenic diet is a low-carb, high-fat way of eating that shifts your body into a metabolic state called ketosis. In ketosis, your body burns fat for fuel instead of glucose. To successfully achieve and remain in ketosis, there are some essential guidelines to follow:

## Carb Restriction

Limiting your total carbohydrate intake to 20-30 net grams per day is typically required to reach ketosis.

Focus on low-carb vegetable sources and avoid grains, legumes, starchy vegetables and sugary foods.

Increase Healthy Fats

On a keto diet, 60-80% of your calories will come from healthy fat sources like avocados, olive oil, nuts, seeds, fatty fish, eggs, and meat. Fat is satiating and your new primary energy source.

## Moderate Protein

While protein is necessary to build and maintain muscle, consuming too much can kick you out of ketosis. Aim for 0.6-1.0

grams of protein per pound of lean body mass.

## Stay Hydrated

Ketosis has a natural diuretic effect, so it's crucial to drink plenty of fluids like water, broths, unsweetened seltzers and herbal teas. Adding electrolytes can help with hydration.

## Test Ketone Levels

Using urine, breath or blood ketone meters can help you determine if you've reached ketosis and adjust your macros accordingly. Optimal ketosis is 0.5-3.0 mmol/L on a blood meter.

## Be Mindful of Micronutrients

While restricting carbs, focus on nutrient-dense protein and veggie sources to avoid potential micronutrient deficiencies. Supplements may also be beneficial.

## Practice Intermittent Fasting

Methods like 16/8 or OMAD (one meal a day) fasting can help induce and maintain ketosis more efficiently when combined with keto.

By sticking to these core principles of restricted carbs, increased healthy fats, moderate protein and staying hydrated, you can successfully follow a ketogenic lifestyle.

Be patient as it can take 1-2 weeks to become fully fat adapted.

# Understanding Inflammation

Inflammation is the body's natural response to protect itself against harm. It is a biological "defense mode" that the immune system initiates when it detects anything potentially dangerous like an infection, injury, or toxin.

Acute inflammation presents itself through familiar symptoms like redness, swelling, heat, and pain around the affected area.

This is a normal - and even necessary - short-term response as the immune system sends extra nourishment and defense to the site via increased blood flow.

Once the harmful source is neutralized or the injury heals, the inflammation should subside.

However, problems arise when inflammation persists long-term with no external cause, resulting in chronic inflammation.

Unlike acute inflammation, chronic inflammation frequently occurs internally without obvious symptoms. This low-grade but consistent inflammation can last for months or even years, damaging healthy cells and tissues.

The most common causes of chronic inflammation include:

Autoimmune disorders like rheumatoid arthritis or lupus where the immune system attacks healthy tissue
Long-term exposure to toxins like pollution or cigarette smoke
Poor diet high in processed foods, unhealthy fats, sugar, etc.
Chronic stress resulting in immune deregulation

Obesity and excess visceral fat
Lack of exercise and sedentary lifestyle

Over time, chronic inflammation increases oxidative stress and has been linked to nearly every major disease including cancer, heart disease, Alzheimer's, diabetes, arthritis, inflammatory bowel diseases, depression, and more. Getting inflammation under control through diet, exercise, stress management and other lifestyle factors is absolutely essential for optimal health.

Understanding the causes, effects, and underlying mechanisms of inflammation is the first step in being able to tackle it effectively through an anti-inflammatory nutrition plan and lifestyle adjustments.

## Anti-Inflammatory Diet

Chronic inflammation has been linked to a wide range of diseases and conditions including rheumatoid arthritis, inflammatory bowel diseases, cancer, heart disease, diabetes, Alzheimer's and more.

While short-term inflammation is a normal

immune response, long-term or chronic inflammation can damage healthy cells and tissues.

One of the most powerful tools we have to reduce chronic inflammation is our diet. An anti-inflammatory diet focuses on nutrient-dense whole foods that can help lower and regulate inflammation levels in the body.
The core principles include:

### Eat Plenty of Antioxidants

Colorful fruits and vegetables like berries, leafy greens, beets, and oranges provide antioxidants that neutralize free radicals that trigger inflammation.

### Focus on Healthy Fats

Omega-3 fatty acids found in fatty fish, walnuts, flax and chia seeds have anti-inflammatory properties. Extra virgin olive oil is also anti-inflammatory.

### Get Enough Fiber

Foods high in fiber like vegetables, fruits, legumes, nuts and seeds help reduce inflammation by feeding beneficial gut bacteria.

## Load Up on Spices/Herbs

Turmeric, ginger, cinnamon, cayenne and other spices/herbs contain potent anti-inflammatory compounds.

## Limit Processed Foods

Highly processed foods often contain inflammatory ingredients like refined carbs, unhealthy fats, sugar and additives.

## Stay Hydrated

Proper hydration allows cells to detox and remove inflammatory compounds.

Manage Stress
Chronic stress leads to inflammation, so strategies like exercise, meditation and getting quality sleep are key.

By focusing your diet on nutrient-dense anti-inflammatory foods while limiting inflammatory triggers, you can help regulate inflammation levels and reduce disease risk. Combined with the ketogenic approach of carb restriction, this diet maximizes anti-inflammatory benefits.

## Foods to Avoid or Limit

Refined carbohydrates (white bread, pastries, pasta, etc.)
Fried foods and unhealthy fats (vegetable oils, margarine, lard)
Sugary beverages (soda, juices)
Red and processed meats
Artificial additives and preservatives
Excessive alcohol intake

These foods may trigger inflammation through various mechanisms like causing an imbalance in omega-6 and omega-3 fatty acids, spiking blood sugar levels, or irritating the gut lining. They provide little nutritional value as well.
Music OK
On the other hand, some of the most anti-inflammatory foods to prioritize include:

## Top Anti-Inflammatory Foods

Fatty fish like salmon, mackerel, sardines
Green leafy vegetables like spinach, kale, collards

Nuts like almonds and walnuts
Berries like blueberries and raspberries
Olive oil and avocados
Green tea
Peppers, mushrooms, tomatoes
Turmeric, ginger, green herbs

These foods are rich in antioxidants like polyphenols that fight oxidative stress, as well as fats like omega-3s that regulate inflammation. Focusing on a variety of these anti-inflammatory superstars can help lower inflammation significantly.

Overall, adopting an anti-inflammatory diet means prioritizing nutrient-dense, minimally-processed plant and animal foods while limiting pro-inflammatory items. This dietary pattern complements the ketogenic approach beautifully for managing chronic inflammation.

## Exercise for Reducing Inflammation

While diet is crucial for managing inflammation, exercise also plays an important role. Regular physical activity can help reduce inflammatory markers and provide numerous other health benefits.

## The Anti-Inflammatory Effects of Exercise

When you exercise, your muscle tissues release anti-inflammatory substances called cytokines into your bloodstream.

These cytokines help counteract inflammation and promote an anti-inflammatory environment throughout the body. Exercise also increases antioxidant production to neutralize free radicals that drive inflammation.

Additionally, maintaining a healthy weight through exercise prevents inflammation triggered by excess body fat, especially visceral abdominal fat.
Chronic overweight and obesity are strongly linked to heightened inflammation.

### Recommended Exercise Types

While any exercise is better than none, certain types may be particularly beneficial for reducing inflammation:

### Aerobic Exercise

Activities like brisk walking, running, cycling or swimming get your heart pumping and increase blood flow to deliver anti-inflammatory substances throughout the body.

**Strength Training**

Resistance exercise like weightlifting causes a short-term inflammatory response to repair muscle fibers, but has an overall anti-inflammatory effect long-term.

**Yoga/Stretching**

The breathing, mindfulness and stretching involved in yoga and other flexibility exercises can lower inflammation by reducing stress hormones.

High Intensity Interval Training (HIIT)
Short bursts of vigorous cardio followed by lower intensity recovery periods produce an acute anti-inflammatory response post-exercise.

Incorporating a mix of these different exercise modalities 3-5 times per week is ideal. Start slow if you're new to exercise to avoid excess inflammation from over-training initially.

In addition to directly impacting inflammation, exercise provides benefits like improved sleep, mood, and stress management which also play a role in regulating inflammation levels.

Making regular physical activity a lifestyle habit is key for maximizing anti-inflammatory effects.

# Combined Keto and Anti-inflammatory Meal Plans

By now, you understand the principles behind both the ketogenic diet and an anti-inflammatory nutritional approach. While they have some overlap, combining these two ways of eating allows you to maximize the health benefits of reducing inflammation while achieving all the other advantages of nutritional ketosis.

This section provides a 30-day meal plan along with a wide variety of delicious recipes that adhere to both the keto and anti-inflammatory diet guidelines. These meals emphasize nutrient-dense whole foods while limiting potential inflammatory triggers.

## 30-Day Keto Anti-Inflammatory Meal Plan

To take the guesswork out of what to eat, we've provided a full 30-day meal plan that is low in carbs to maintain ketosis while also prioritizing anti-inflammatory ingredients. Each day includes three meals and a couple of snack options.

This meal plan offers a good mix of comforting classics and internationally-inspired flavors to keep you satisfied without getting bored. You'll find lots of healthy fats, clean proteins, low-carb veggies, and antioxidant-rich herbs and spices in each recipe.

A comprehensive shopping list is provided to make meal prepping easy.

There are also suggestions for swaps or substitutions based on your personal preferences.

Sample meal plan days include:

Keto Saag Paneer with Cauliflower Rice
Salmon Veggie Packets with Lemon Dill Butter
Keto Burgers with Avocado and Keto Fries
Coconut Curry Chicken
Mediterranean Lamb Bowls

And many more nutrient-packed, anti-inflammatory friendly options for breakfast, lunch, dinner, smoothies, and snacks!

## Recipes

To complement the 30-day plan, over 75 keto anti-inflammatory recipes are included for every meal and course so you can build your own custom meal plans moving forward:

Breakfast: Baked Avocado Eggs, Keto Smoothies
Salads & Sides: Keto Cauliflower Potato Salad, Garlic Greens
Mains: Lemon Dill Salmon, Chicken Fajita Bowls, Keto Cabbage Rolls

Soups & Stews: Golden Turmeric Chicken Soup, Chili Colorado
Snacks & Desserts: Keto Avocado Brownies, Anti-Inflammatory Trail Mix

All recipes contain the macros per serving as well as helpful tips to minimize prep time and make swaps.

With so many varied and flavorful options, you'll have all you need to sustain the keto anti-inflammatory lifestyle long-term.

Whether you follow the full 30-day plan or mix-and-match your own meals, this section equips you with everything required to combat inflammation through nutrient-dense keto eating.

## 30-Day Meal Plan

This comprehensive 30-day plan combines the principles of the ketogenic diet with an anti-inflammatory nutritional approach.

Each day provides three meals and a couple of snack options that are low in carbs to maintain ketosis while emphasizing nutrient-dense, anti-inflammatory ingredients like healthy fats, clean proteins, antioxidant-rich produce, and anti-inflammatory herbs and spices.

## Week 1

**Day** 1: Keto Frittata with Sauteed Greens, Salmon Avocado Boats, Keto Pulled Pork with Cauliflower Mash

**Day** 2: Coconut Flour Pancakes with Berry Topping, Loaded Avocado Salad, Lemongrass Thai Curry Meatballs

**Day** 3: Keto Smoothie, Steak Fajita Bowl, Keto Cabbage Rolls

**Day** 4: Baked Avocado Eggs, Chicken BLT Salad, Slow Cooker Beef Curry

**Day** 5: Keto Breakfast Sandwich, Zucchini Rollatini, Creamy Turmeric Chicken Skillet

**Day** 6: Keto Overnight "Oats", Mediterranean Lamb Bowls, 5-Ingredient Stuffed Peppers

**Day** 7: Egg Muffin Cups, Cauliflower Potato

Salad, Creamy Garlic Shrimp

## Week 2

**Day** 8: Coconut Chia Pudding, Loaded Bacon Avocado Salad, Meatball Parmesan with Zucchini Noodles

**Day** 9: Keto Green Smoothie, Salmon Veggie Packets, Keto Broccoli Cheese Soup

**Day** 10: Keto Cream Cheese Pancakes, Keto Chicken BLT Wraps, Beef Stir Fry with Cauliflower Rice

**Day** 11: Keto Ham and Cheese Frittata, Ahi Tuna Poke Bowl, Slow Cooker Pork Carnitas

...

An appendix with a master grocery list for the full 30 days as well as suggestions for easy meal prep, swaps and substitutions is also included to set you up for success on this plan.

With the combined benefits of nutritional ketosis and anti-inflammatory nutrition, you'll feel energized, reduce inflammation, and potentially experience health improvements across the board.

## Week 3

**Day** 15: Keto Coconut Flour Waffles, Greek Salad Skewers, Broccoli Cheddar Keto Soup

**Day** 16: Keto Smoothie Bowl, Crispy Chicken Salad, Mediterranean Lamb Skewers

**Day** 17: Keto Breakfast Taco Cups, Steak Fajita Lettuce Wraps, Lemon Garlic Sardines

**Day** 18: Baked Avocado Egg Boats, Keto BLT Salad, Creamy Tuscan Shrimp

**Day** 19: Keto Frittata, Spicy Tuna Cucumber Boats, Slow Cooker Mexican Beef Bowl

**Day** 20: Coconut Chia Pudding, Zucchini Rollatini, Keto Butter Chicken

**Day** 21: Ham & Cheese Egg Cups, Anti-Inflammatory Trail Mix, Creamy Garlic Shrimp over Zoodles

## Week 4

**Day** 22: Keto Green Smoothie, Loaded

Avocado Turkey Salad, Coconut Curry Chicken

**Day** 23: Keto Tortilla Bowl, Salmon Avocado Salad, Keto Stuffed Peppers

**Day** 24: Overnight Keto Oats, Greek Salad Skewers, Slow Cooker Beef Bone Broth Soup

**Day** 25: Cream Cheese Pancakes, Steak & Avocado Salad, Lemongrass Meatballs over Cauli-Rice

**Day** 26: Keto Breakfast Sandwich, Keto BLT Wraps, Golden Turmeric Chicken Soup

**Day** 27: Egg Muffin Cups, Broccoli Salad, Keto Cabbage Rolls

**Day** 28: Baked Avocado Eggs, Tuna Salad Lettuce Wraps, Creamy Garlic Shrimp Zoodles

## Week 5

**Day** 29: Coconut Flour Waffles, Salsa Verde Chicken Salad, Pork Carnitas Lettuce Cups

**Day** 30: Keto Smoothie Bowl, Keto Chili Colorado, Keto Avocado Brownies

This provides a balanced mix of flavors and ingredients to cover all your meals for a full 30 days on a ketogenic and anti-inflammatory nutrition plan.

Recipes emphasize clean proteins, healthy fats, low-carb veggies, and antioxidant-rich herbs and spices.

Be sure to drink plenty of fluids and consider adding electrolyte supplements on keto. You can also do simple swaps of proteins or produce to suit your tastes.

The key is setting yourself up for success by having a structured plan that aligns with your dietary goals.

# Chapter 2

# Recipes

# Section

# Breakfast

## Baked Avocado Eggs
**Prep Time: 10 minutes Cook Time: 20 minutes Total Time: 30 minutes Servings: 2**

A deliciously creamy and satisfying way to start your day! These baked avocado boats are filled with egg and topped with fresh herbs, cheese, and anti-inflammatory extras like tomatoes.

## Ingredients:

2 medium ripe avocados 4 eggs 2 tablespoons crumbled feta or goat cheese 2 tablespoons diced tomatoes 1 tablespoon chopped fresh basil or parsley 1/4 teaspoon garlic powder 1/4 teaspoon red pepper flakes (optional) Salt and pepper to taste

## Instructions:

1. Preheat oven to 425°F.
2. Cut the avocados in half lengthwise

and remove the pit. Scoop out about 1-2 tablespoons from the center of each avocado half to make a little more room for the egg.

3. Place the avocado halves in a small baking dish or on a parchment-lined baking sheet.
4. Crack an egg into each avocado half, trying not to overflow the edges.
5. Top each stuffed avocado with feta/goat cheese, diced tomatoes, fresh herbs, garlic powder, red pepper flakes if using, and salt & pepper.
6. Bake for 15-20 minutes until the egg whites are completely set but the yolks are still a bit runny.
7. Carefully remove from oven and allow to cool slightly before serving.

**Nutrition per serving (2 avocado halves): Calories: 425 Total Fat: 36g Total Carbs: 15g Fiber: 11g Net Carbs: 4g Protein: 15g**

This filling breakfast packs healthy fats from the avocado and egg, plus anti-inflammatory benefits from fresh herbs, tomatoes and spices.

It's a delicious way to fuel up in the morning! Enjoy it as is or serve with a side salad.

Notes:

- Can sub dairy-free cheese for feta if needed
- Top with extras like bacon, salsa, or hot sauce if desired
- Keep avocado halves upright in the baking dish to prevent spilling

**Keto Coconut Flour Waffles**

**Prep Time: 10 mins Cook Time: 15 mins Total Time:                25                mins**
**Servings: 4 waffles**

Ingredients:

- 1/2 cup coconut flour
- 1/4 cup almond flour
- 1 tsp baking powder
- 1/4 tsp salt
- 4 eggs
- 1/4 cup coconut oil, melted
- 1/4 cup unsweetened almond milk
- 1 tsp vanilla extract

**Instructions**:

1. In a bowl, whisk together coconut

flour, almond flour, baking powder and salt.
2. In another bowl, beat eggs then whisk in coconut oil, almond milk and vanilla.
3. Pour wet into dry and mix until fully combined, let batter rest 5 mins.
4. Scoop 1/4 of batter onto preheated waffle iron and cook 5-7 mins until golden.

**Nutrition per waffle: Calories: 285 Fat: 23g Carbs: 12g Fiber: 6g Net Carbs: 6g Protein: 8g**

## Keto Cream Cheese Pancakes

**Prep Time: 5 mins Cook Time: 10 mins Total Time: 15 mins Servings: 8 pancakes**

### Ingredients:

- 4 oz cream cheese, softened
- 4 eggs
- 1 tsp vanilla
- 1/2 tsp cinnamon
- 1/4 tsp baking powder
- 2 tbsp almond flour (or coconut)
- Butter or oil for cooking

### Instructions:

1. In a blender, blend together cream cheese, eggs, vanilla, cinnamon and baking powder until smooth.
2. Pour in almond flour and pulse to incorporate.
3. Heat skillet or griddle over medium heat with butter or oil.
4. Pour out 1/4 cup portions of batter onto hot surface and cook 2-3 mins per side.

Nutrition per 2 pancakes: Calories: 222 Fat: 20g Carbs: 4g Fiber: 1g Net Carbs: 3g Protein: 8g

## Keto Green Smoothie Bowl

Prep Time: 10 mins Total Time: 10 mins Servings: 1

### Ingredients:

- 1 cup unsweetened almond milk
- 1/2 avocado
- 1 cup spinach
- 1/2 cup frozen cauliflower rice
- 2 tbsp almond butter
- 1 scoop vanilla protein powder
- 1 tbsp chia seeds
- 1 tsp cinnamon

**Instructions**:

1. Add all ingredients to a blender and blend until very smooth and creamy.
2. Pour into a bowl and top with desired low-carb toppings like nuts, seeds, berries, or shredded coconut.

**Nutrition:** **Calories:** **485**
**Fat: 36g Carbs: 18g Fiber: 13g Net Carbs: 5g Protein: 29g**

## Keto Ham & Cheese Frittata Muffins

**Prep Time: 10 mins Cook Time: 25 mins Total Time: 35 mins Servings: 12 muffins**

### Ingredients:

- 10 eggs
- 1/4 cup heavy cream
- 1 cup shredded cheddar
- 1/2 cup diced ham
- 1/4 cup sliced green onion
- 1 tsp dried parsley
- 1/2 tsp salt
- 1/4 tsp black pepper

**Instructions:**

1. Preheat oven to 375°F and grease a

muffin tin.
2. In a bowl, whisk together eggs, cream,
   1/2 cup cheese, ham, onion, parsley,
   salt and pepper.
3. Pour egg mixture evenly into muffin
   cups, sprinkle with remaining 1/2 cup
   cheese.
4. Bake 20-25 mins until puffy and
   centers are set.
5. Let cool 5 mins before removing from
   tin.

**Nutrition per muffin: Calories: 140 Fat: 10g Carbs: 1g Fiber: 0g Net Carbs: 1g Protein: 11g**

## Coconut Flour Biscuits with Sausage Gravy

**Prep Time: 10 mins Cook Time: 15 mins Total Time: 25 mins Servings: 6 biscuits**

For the biscuits:

- 1/2 cup coconut flour
- 1/4 tsp salt
- 1/2 tsp baking powder
- 3 eggs
- 3 tbsp coconut oil, melted
- 2 tbsp unsweetened almond milk

For the gravy:

- 1 lb ground breakfast sausage
- 2 tbsp butter
- 2 cups unsweetened almond milk
- 2 tbsp coconut flour
- 1/2 tsp black pepper
- 1/4 tsp xanthan gum (optional)

**Instructions:**

1. For biscuits, whisk flour, salt and baking powder. Mix in eggs, coconut oil and milk until combined.
2. Drop spoonfuls of dough onto parchment lined baking sheet and bake at 375°F for 14-16 mins.
3. For gravy, cook sausage in a skillet over medium, drain excess fat. Add butter, milk and coconut flour and whisk constantly until thickened to desired consistency. Add pepper and xanthan gum if using.
4. Serve sausage gravy over biscuits.

**Nutrition per biscuit with 1/6th gravy: Calories: 383 Fat: 35g Carbs: 7g Fiber: 3g Net Carbs: 4g Protein: 16g**

# Keto Smoothie

**Keto Green Smoothie**

**Prep Time: 5 mins Cook Time: 0 mins
Servings: 1**

**Ingredients:**

- 1 cup unsweetened almond milk
- 1 cup baby spinach
- 1/2 avocado
- 1/2 cup frozen cauliflower rice
- 1 scoop unflavored protein powder
- 1 tbsp nut butter
- 1 tbsp chia seeds
- 1/2 tsp cinnamon
- Stevia or monk fruit to taste (optional)

## Instructions:

1. Add all ingredients to a blender and blend until completely smooth.
2. Taste and adjust sweetener if desired.
3. Pour into a glass and enjoy!

**Nutrition per serving: Calories: 427, Fat: 34g, Carbs: 15g, Fiber: 12g, Protein: 22g**

## Keto Peanut Butter Smoothie

**Prep Time: 5 mins
Cook Time: 0 mins Servings: 1**

**Ingredients**:

- 1 cup unsweetened almond milk
- 2 tbsp natural peanut butter
- 1 scoop vanilla protein powder
- 1 tbsp cocoa powder
- 1/4 tsp cinnamon
- 1-2 tbsp erythritol (optional)
- 1 cup ice cubes

## Instructions:

1. Add all ingredients to a blender and blend until thick and creamy.
2. Taste and adjust sweetener if needed.
3. Pour into a glass and enjoy!

**Nutrition per serving: Calories: 380, Fat: 23g, Carbs: 10g, Fiber: 5g, Protein: 35g**

## Keto Coconut Mango Smoothie

**Prep Time: 5 mins Cook Time: 0 mins Servings: 1**

**Ingredients**:

- 1/2 cup unsweetened coconut milk
- 1/2 cup frozen mango chunks
- 1/4 avocado
- 1 scoop vanilla protein powder
- 1 tbsp coconut butter
- 1 tsp lemon juice
- Stevia or monk fruit to taste (optional)

**Instructions**:

1. Add all ingredients to a blender and blend until completely smooth.
2. Adjust sweetener to taste if desired.
3. Pour into a glass and enjoy!

**Nutrition per serving: Calories: 375, Fat: 22g, Carbs: 16g, Fiber: 7g, Protein: 25g**

## Keto Mocha Smoothie

**Prep Time: 5 mins Cook Time: 0 mins Servings: 1**

**Ingredients**:

- 1 cup unsweetened almond milk
- 1 tbsp cocoa powder
- 1 shot hot coffee or espresso
- 1 scoop chocolate protein powder
- 1 tbsp MCT oil or coconut oil
- 1-2 tbsp erythritol (optional)
- 1/4 tsp vanilla extract
- Pinch of sea salt
- Handful of ice cubes

## Instructions:

1. Add all ingredients to a blender and blend until smooth and frothy.
2. Taste and adjust sweetener if needed.
3. Pour into a glass and enjoy!

**Nutrition per serving: Calories: 292, Fat: 20g, Carbs: 8g, Fiber: 5g, Protein: 24g**

## Keto Strawberry Smoothie

## Prep Time: 5 mins Cook Time: 0 mins Servings: 1

Ingredients:

- 3/4 cup unsweetened almond milk
- 1/2 cup frozen strawberries

- 1/4 avocado
- 1 scoop vanilla protein powder
- 1 tbsp almond butter
- 1 tsp lemon juice
- Stevia or monk fruit to taste (optional)

## Instructions:

1. Add all ingredients to a blender and blend until smooth.
2. Taste and adjust sweetener if desired.
3. Pour into a glass and enjoy!

**Nutrition Per Serving: Calories 389, Fat 27g, Carbs 14g, Fiber 8g, Protein 26g**

## Keto Turmeric Smoothie

## Prep Time: 5 mins Cook Time: 0 mins Servings: 1

## Ingredients:

- 1 cup unsweetened coconut milk
- 1/2 frozen banana
- 1 tbsp almond butter
- 1 tsp turmeric
- 1 tsp grated ginger
- 1 tbsp MCT oil or coconut oil

- Pinch of black pepper
- Stevia or monk fruit to taste (optional)

## Instructions:

1. Add all ingredients to a blender and blend until completely smooth.
2. Taste and adjust sweetener if desired.
3. Pour into a glass and enjoy!

**Nutrition Per Serving: Calories 366, Fat 31g, Carbs 13g, Fiber 5g, Protein 7g**

## Keto Matcha Smoothie

## Prep Time: 5 mins Cook Time: 0 mins Servings: 1

## Ingredients:

- 1 cup unsweetened almond milk
- 1 scoop unflavored or vanilla protein powder
- 1 tsp matcha green tea powder
- 1/2 avocado
- 1 tbsp almond butter
- 1 tbsp chia seeds
- Stevia or monk fruit to taste (optional)

## Instructions:

1. Add all ingredients except chia seeds to a blender and blend until completely smooth.
2. Stir in the chia seeds.
3. Taste and adjust sweetener if desired.
4. Pour into a glass and enjoy!

**Nutrition Per Serving: Calories 413, Fat 30g, Carbs 14g, Fiber 12g, Protein 24g**

## Keto Golden Milk Smoothie

## Prep Time: 5 mins Cook Time: 0 mins Servings: 1

### Ingredients:

- 1 cup unsweetened almond milk
- 1/2 cup full-fat coconut milk
- 1 tbsp MCT oil or coconut oil
- 1/2 tsp ground turmeric
- 1/2 tsp ground ginger
- 1/4 tsp ground cinnamon
- 1/4 tsp vanilla extract
- Stevia or monk fruit to taste (optional)

### Instructions:

1. Add all ingredients to a blender and

blend until completely smooth.
2. Taste and adjust sweetener if desired.
3. Pour into a glass and enjoy!

**Nutrition Per Serving: Calories 330, Fat 32g, Carbs 5g, Fiber 2g, Protein 2g**

## Keto Peppermint Mocha Smoothie

**Prep Time: 5 mins Cook Time: 0 mins Servings: 1**

### Ingredients:

- 1 cup unsweetened almond milk
- 1 tbsp cocoa powder
- 1 shot hot coffee or espresso
- 1 scoop chocolate protein powder
- 1 tbsp MCT oil or coconut oil
- 1/4 tsp peppermint extract
- 1-2 tbsp erythritol (optional)

### Instructions:

1. Add all ingredients to a blender and blend until smooth and frothy.
2. Taste and adjust sweetener if needed.
3. Pour into a glass and enjoy!

**Nutrition Per Serving: Calories 307, Fat 21g,**

**Carbs 9g, Fiber 5g, Protein 24g**

## Keto Chocolate Avocado Smoothie

## Prep Time: 5 mins Cook Time: 0 mins Servings: 1

### Ingredients:

- 1 cup unsweetened almond milk
- 1/2 avocado
- 2 tbsp cocoa powder
- 1 scoop chocolate protein powder
- 1 tbsp almond butter
- 1 tsp vanilla extract
- Stevia or monk fruit to taste (optional)
- Handful of ice

### Instructions:

1. Add all ingredients to a blender and blend until completely smooth.
2. Taste and adjust sweetener if desired.
3. Pour into a glass and enjoy!

**Nutrition Per Serving: Calories 469, Fat 36g, Carbs 17g, Fiber 11g, Protein 27g**

# Keto Blueberry Cheesecake Smoothie

## Prep Time: 5 mins Cook Time: 0 mins Servings: 1

### Ingredients:

- 1 cup unsweetened almond milk
- 1/2 cup frozen blueberries
- 1/4 cup full-fat cream cheese
- 1 scoop vanilla protein powder
- 1 tsp lemon juice
- 1/4 tsp vanilla extract
- Stevia or monk fruit to taste (optional)

### Instructions:

1. Add all ingredients to a blender and blend until completely smooth.
2. Taste and adjust sweetener if desired.
3. Pour into a glass and enjoy!

**Nutrition Per Serving: Calories 388, Fat 24g, Carbs 14g, Fiber 5g, Protein 31g**

# Keto Chai Smoothie

## Prep Time: 5 mins Cook Time: 0 mins Servings: 1

**Ingredients**:

- 1 cup unsweetened almond milk
- 1/4 cup full-fat coconut milk
- 1 scoop vanilla protein powder
- 1 tsp chai spice mix
- 1 tbsp almond butter
- 1 tbsp MCT oil or coconut oil
- Stevia or monk fruit to taste (optional)
- Handful of ice

## Instructions:

1. Add all ingredients to a blender and blend until smooth.
2. Taste and adjust sweetener if desired.
3. Pour into a glass and enjoy!

**Nutrition Per Serving: Calories 432, Fat 35g, Carbs 10g, Fiber 5g, Protein 25g**

## Keto Pumpkin Spice Smoothie

## Prep Time: 5 mins Cook Time: 0 mins Servings: 1

## Ingredients:

- 1 cup unsweetened almond milk
- 1/2 cup canned pumpkin puree

- 1 scoop vanilla protein powder
- 1 tbsp almond butter
- 1 tsp pumpkin pie spice
- 1/4 tsp vanilla extract
- Stevia or monk fruit to taste (optional)
- Handful of ice

## Instructions:

1. Add all ingredients to a blender and blend until completely smooth.
2. Taste and adjust sweetener if desired.
3. Pour into a glass and enjoy!

**Nutrition Per Serving: Calories 319, Fat 19g, Carbs 14g, Fiber 8g, Protein 27g**


## Keto Coconut Acai Smoothie

## Prep Time: 5 mins Cook Time: 0 mins Servings: 1

## Ingredients:

- 1 cup unsweetened coconut milk
- 1/2 cup frozen acai puree
- 1/4 avocado
- 1 scoop vanilla protein powder
- 1 tbsp coconut butter

- 1 tbsp chia seeds
- Stevia or monk fruit to taste (optional)

## Instructions:

1. Add all ingredients except chia seeds to a blender and blend until smooth.
2. Stir in the chia seeds.
3. Taste and adjust sweetener if desired.
4. Pour into a glass and enjoy!

**Nutrition Per Serving: Calories 474, Fat 35g, Carbs 19g, Fiber 14g, Protein 22g**

## Keto Cinnamon Roll Smoothie

## Prep Time: 5 mins Cook Time: 0 mins Servings: 1

## Ingredients:

- 1 cup unsweetened almond milk
- 1/2 cup cottage cheese
- 1 scoop vanilla protein powder
- 1 tbsp almond butter
- 1 tsp ground cinnamon
- 1/4 tsp vanilla extract
- Pinch of nutmeg
- Stevia or monk fruit to taste (optional)

**Instructions**:

1. Add all ingredients to a blender and blend until completely smooth.
2. Taste and adjust sweetener if desired.
3. Pour into a glass and enjoy!

**Nutrition Per Serving: Calories 391, Fat 24g, Carbs 10g, Fiber 4g, Protein 37g**

## Keto Raspberry Cheesecake Smoothie

## Prep Time: 5 mins Cook Time: 0 mins Servings: 1

### Ingredients:

- 3/4 cup unsweetened almond milk
- 1/2 cup frozen raspberries
- 1/4 cup full-fat cream cheese
- 1 scoop vanilla protein powder
- 1 tsp lemon juice
- Stevia or monk fruit to taste (optional)

### Instructions:

1. Add all ingredients to a blender and blend until completely smooth.
2. Taste and adjust sweetener if desired.
3. Pour into a glass and enjoy!

Nutrition Per Serving: Calories 372, Fat 22g, Carbs 13g, Fiber 7g, Protein 31g

## Keto Pecan Pie Smoothie

## Prep Time: 5 mins Cook Time: 0 mins Servings: 1

### Ingredients:

- 1 cup unsweetened almond milk
- 1/4 cup pecans
- 1 scoop vanilla protein powder
- 1 tbsp almond butter
- 1 tsp ground cinnamon
- 1/4 tsp vanilla extract
- Pinch of nutmeg
- Stevia or monk fruit to taste (optional)

### Instructions:

1. Add all ingredients to a blender and blend until completely smooth.
2. Taste and adjust sweetener if desired.
3. Pour into a glass and enjoy!

Nutrition Per Serving: Calories 495, Fat 38g, Carbs 13g, Fiber 6g, Protein 29g

# Keto Pineapple Smoothie

## Prep Time: 5 mins Cook Time: 0 mins Servings: 1

### Ingredients:

- 1 cup unsweetened coconut milk
- 1/2 cup frozen pineapple chunks
- 1/4 avocado
- 1 scoop vanilla protein powder
- 1 tbsp MCT oil or coconut oil
- Stevia or monk fruit to taste (optional)
- Squeeze of lime juice

## Instructions:

1. Add all ingredients to a blender and blend until completely smooth.
2. Taste and adjust sweetener if desired.
3. Pour into a glass and enjoy!

**Nutrition Per Serving: Calories 412, Fat 28g, Carbs 16g, Fiber 7g, Protein 23g**


# Keto Almond Butter Cup Smoothie

## Prep Time: 5 mins Cook Time: 0 mins Servings: 1

## Ingredients:

- 1 cup unsweetened almond milk
- 2 tbsp natural almond butter
- 2 tbsp cocoa powder
- 1 scoop chocolate protein powder
- 1/4 tsp vanilla extract
- Pinch of sea salt
- Stevia or monk fruit to taste (optional)
- Handful of ice

## Instructions:

1. Add all ingredients to a blender and blend until smooth.
2. Taste and adjust sweetener if desired.
3. Pour into a glass and enjoy!

**Nutrition Per Serving: Calories 391, Fat 27g, Carbs 12g, Fiber 7g, Protein 30g**

# Salads and Sides

## Avocado Keto Green Goddess Dressing

**Prep Time: 10 mins Total Time: 10 mins Servings: 8 (2 tbsp per serving)**

### Ingredients:

- 1 avocado
- 1/2 cup olive oil
- 1/4 cup fresh parsley
- 2 tbsp fresh dill
- 2 tbsp lemon juice
- 1 clove garlic
- 1 tsp Dijon mustard
- 1/2 tsp salt
- 1/4 tsp black pepper

### Instructions:

1. Add all ingredients to a blender or food processor.
2. Blend until completely smooth and creamy.
3. Taste and adjust seasoning as needed.
4. Store leftover dressing in the fridge for up to 5 days.

Nutrition per 2 tbsp serving: Calories: 138 Fat: 14g Carbs: 2g Fiber: 1g Net Carbs: 1g Protein: 1g

## Garlic Greens with Lemon and Bacon

Prep Time: 10 mins Cook Time: 10 mins Total Time: 20 mins Servings: 4

**Ingredients**:

- 8 oz baby spinach
- 8 oz kale, stems removed and chopped
- 4 slices bacon, diced
- 2 cloves garlic, minced
- 1 tbsp olive oil
- 2 tbsp lemon juice
- 1/4 tsp red pepper flakes
- Salt and pepper to taste

**Instructions**:

1. In a large skillet, cook diced bacon over medium-high until crispy. Remove to a plate, keeping bacon fat in pan.
2. Add olive oil and garlic to the pan and sauté for 1 minute until fragrant.
3. Add in the spinach and kale. Toss frequently until wilted down, about 3-4 minutes.
4. Remove pan from heat and stir in lemon juice, red pepper flakes and cooked bacon. Season with salt and pepper to taste.
5. Serve greens immediately while hot.

**Nutrition per Serving (1/4th recipe): Calories: 150 Fat: 12g Carbs: 6g Fiber: 2g Net Carbs: 4g Protein: 6g**

## Spicy Keto Cauliflower Salad

**Prep Time: 15 mins**
**Total Time: 15 mins Servings: 6**

### Ingredients:

- 1 head cauliflower, cut into florets
- 1 jalapeño, seeded and diced
- 1/2 cup chopped cilantro
- 2 green onions, sliced
- 1/2 cup crumbled cotija or feta cheese
- 2 tbsp olive oil
- 2 tbsp red wine vinegar
- 1 tbsp lime juice
- 1 tsp cumin
- 1/4 tsp garlic powder
- 1/4 tsp chili powder
- Salt and pepper to taste

### Instructions:

1. In a large bowl, add cauliflower florets, jalapeño, cilantro, green onions and cheese.
2. In a small bowl, whisk together olive oil, vinegar, lime juice and spices.
3. Pour dressing over cauliflower mixture and toss to coat evenly.

4. Season with salt and pepper to taste.
5. Let sit 10-15 minutes before serving to allow flavors to meld.

**Nutrition per Serving (1/6th recipe): Calories: 126 Fat: 9g Carbs: 6g Fiber: 3g Net Carbs: 3g Protein: 4g**

## Loaded Cauliflower "Potato" Salad

**Prep Time: 20 mins Cook Time: 10 mins Total Time: 30 mins Servings: 6**

### Ingredients:

- 1 medium head cauliflower, cut into florets (6 cups)
- 1/4 cup diced celery
- 1/4 cup diced red onion
- 2 tbsp chopped fresh dill
- 2 tbsp chopped fresh parsley
- 1/2 cup avocado mayo
- 2 tbsp lemon juice
- 1 tbsp Dijon mustard
- 1 tsp apple cider vinegar
- 1 clove garlic, minced
- 1 tsp dried dill
- 1/2 tsp salt
- 1/4 tsp black pepper

**Instructions**:

1. Bring a pot of salted water to a boil. Cook cauliflower 5-7 mins until tender. Drain and rinse with cold water.
2. In a bowl, whisk together mayo, lemon juice, mustard, vinegar, garlic, dill, salt and pepper.
3. In a large bowl, combine cauliflower, celery, onion, herbs.
4. Pour dressing over cauliflower and toss to coat.
5. Refrigerate at least 30 mins before serving.

Nutrition per Serving (1/6th recipe): Calories: 210 Fat: 21g Carbs: 5g Fiber: 2g Net Carbs: 3g Protein: 2g

## Zucchini Noodles with Pesto

Prep Time: 15 mins Total Time: 15 mins Servings: 4

**Ingredients**:

- 4 medium zucchini, spiralized into noodles
- 1 cup packed basil leaves
- 1/2 cup olive oil

- 1/4 cup pine nuts or slivered almonds
- 2 cloves garlic
- 1/4 cup grated parmesan
- 1 tbsp lemon juice
- 1/2 tsp salt
- 1/4 tsp pepper

**Instructions**:

1. In a food processor, pulse together the basil, olive oil, nuts, garlic and lemon juice until a rough pesto forms. Transfer to a bowl and stir in parmesan.
2. Add zucchini noodles to a large bowl. Pour pesto over top and toss until fully coated.
3. Season zoodles with salt and pepper.
4. Let sit 5 minutes before serving to allow zoodles to soften slightly.
5. Enjoy zoodles warm, cold or at room temp!

**Nutrition per Serving (1/4th recipe): Calories: 334 Fat: 32g                    Carbs:                    9g Fiber: 2g Net Carbs: 7g Protein: 5g**

## Broccoli Bacon Salad

**Prep Time: 20 mins Total Time: 20 mins Servings: 6**

**Ingredients**:

- 6 cups fresh broccoli florets
- 6 slices bacon, cooked and crumbled
- 1/3 cup diced red onion
- 1/2 cup mayonnaise
- 1 tbsp apple cider vinegar
- 1 tbsp erythritol or monk fruit sweetener
- 1/2 tsp dijon mustard
- 1/4 tsp salt
- 1/8 tsp black pepper

**Instructions**:

1. In a large bowl, combine broccoli florets, crumbled bacon, and red onion.
2. In a small bowl, whisk together mayo, vinegar, sweetener, mustard, salt and pepper.
3. Pour dressing over broccoli mixture and toss until fully coated.
4. Refrigerate for 30 mins before serving to allow flavors to meld.

**Nutrition per Serving (1/6th recipe): Calories: 210 Fat: 19g Carbs: 5g Fiber: 2g Net Carbs: 3g Protein: 4g**

## Crispy Garlic Brussels Sprouts
**Prep          Time:          10          mins**

**Cook Time: 20 mins Total Time: 30 mins Servings: 4**

## Ingredients:

- 1 lb brussels sprouts, halved
- 3 tbsp avocado oil
- 3 cloves garlic, minced
- 1/4 cup grated parmesan
- 1 tsp lemon zest
- 1/2 tsp salt
- 1/4 tsp black pepper

**Instructions:**

1. Preheat oven to 400°F. Toss brussels sprouts with avocado oil on a baking sheet.
2. Roast for 15 mins, shaking pan halfway.
3. Remove from oven and toss brussels with garlic, parmesan, lemon zest, salt and pepper.
4. Return to oven and roast 5 more mins until crispy.

**Nutrition per Serving (1/4th recipe): Calories: 170 Fat: 13g Carbs: 8g Fiber: 3g Net Carbs: 5g Protein: 5g**

**Keto Jalapeño Popper Cauliflower Salad**

**Prep Time: 20 mins Total Time: 20 mins
Servings: 8**

## Ingredients:

- 6 cups cauliflower florets
- 6 slices bacon, cooked and crumbled
- 4 oz cream cheese, softened
- 1/2 cup mayonnaise
- 1/2 cup shredded cheddar
- 2 jalapeños, seeded and diced
- 1 tsp garlic powder
- 1/2 tsp onion powder
- Salt and pepper to taste

**Instructions:**

1. In a large bowl, combine cauliflower florets, crumbled bacon and diced jalapeños.
2. In a small bowl, mix together cream cheese, mayo, cheddar, garlic powder and onion powder.
3. Pour cream cheese mixture over cauliflower and toss until fully coated.
4. Season with salt and pepper to taste.
5. Refrigerate 30 mins before serving.

**Nutrition per Serving (1/8th recipe): Calories: 237 Fat: 22g Carbs: 4g Fiber: 2g Net Carbs: 2g Protein: 5g**

**Keto Buffalo Cauliflower Bites**

**Prep Time: 10 mins Cook Time: 25 mins Total Time: 35 mins Servings: 6**

## Ingredients:

- 6 cups cauliflower florets
- 1/2 cup buffalo sauce
- 1/2 cup almond flour
- 1 tsp garlic powder
- 1 tsp onion powder
- 1/4 tsp salt
- 1/4 tsp black pepper
- 3 eggs, beaten
- 1/2 cup crumbled blue cheese or ranch, for serving

**Instructions:**

1. Preheat oven to 425°F. Toss cauliflower florets with buffalo sauce.
2. In one bowl, mix together almond flour, spices, salt and pepper. In another bowl, beat eggs.
3. Dip each buffalo cauliflower bite first in egg, then in almond flour mixture to coat.
4. Place coated bites on a parchment-lined baking sheet.
5. Bake for 20-25 mins, flipping halfway

through.

6. Serve warm with ranch or crumbled blue cheese for dipping.

Nutrition per Serving (1/6th recipe): Calories: 165 Fat: 9g
Carbs: 9g Fiber: 4g
Net Carbs: 5g Protein: 9g

## Riced Cauliflower Risotto

**Prep Time: 10 mins Cook Time: 20 mins Total Time: 30 mins Servings: 6**

## Ingredients:

- 1 head cauliflower, riced
- 2 tbsp olive oil
- 1/2 cup diced onion
- 2 cloves garlic, minced
- 2 cups chicken or veggie broth
- 1/2 cup parmesan, plus more for topping
- 3 tbsp butter
- 2 tbsp heavy cream
- 2 tbsp chopped parsley
- Salt and pepper to taste

## Instructions:

1. In a large skillet, cook the riced cauliflower over med-high heat for 5-7 mins, stirring frequently, until

cauliflower is lightly browned and tender crisp.

2. In another skillet, heat olive oil over medium heat. Sauté onion for 2 mins then add garlic and cook 1 min more.
3. Add cauliflower rice to onion skillet along with the broth. Simmer for 10 mins, stirring frequently until cauliflower is very tender.
4. Remove from heat and stir in parmesan, butter, cream and parsley. Season with salt and pepper to taste.
5. Serve warm, garnished with more parmesan if desired.

**Nutrition per Serving (1/6th recipe): Calories: 220 Fat: 17g Carbs: 8g Fiber: 3g Net Carbs: 5g Protein: 8g**

# Mains (Poultry, Seafood, Vegetarian)

**Keto Butter Chicken**

**Prep Time: 15 mins Cook Time: 25 mins Total Time: 40 mins Servings: 6**

**Ingredients**:

- 1.5 lbs boneless, skinless chicken thighs, cut into 1-inch pieces
- 2 tbsp butter
- 1 cup crushed tomatoes
- 1 cup full-fat coconut milk
- 2 tsp garam masala
- 1 tsp paprika
- 1 tsp cumin
- 1 tsp salt
- 1/4 tsp cayenne pepper
- 1/4 cup heavy cream
- 2 tbsp chopped cilantro

**Instructions**:

1. In a skillet over medium-high heat, sauté chicken in butter for 5-7 minutes until browned.
2. Add crushed tomatoes, coconut milk, garam masala, paprika, cumin, salt and cayenne. Bring to a simmer.
3. Reduce heat to medium-low and simmer for 15-20 minutes, stirring occasionally, until chicken is cooked through.
4. Remove from heat and stir in heavy cream and cilantro.
5. Serve over cauliflower rice if desired.

Nutrition per Serving (1/6th recipe): Calories: 320 Fat: 21g Carbs: 5g Fiber: 1g Net Carbs: 4g Protein: 28g

## Mediterranean Cod with Roasted Tomatoes

**Prep Time: 10 mins Cook Time: 20 mins Total Time: 30 mins Servings: 4**

### Ingredients:

- 1.5 lbs cod fillets
- 2 cups cherry tomatoes, halved
- 1/4 cup olive oil, divided
- 3 cloves garlic, minced
- 1 tsp dried oregano
- Salt and pepper to taste
- 2 tbsp chopped fresh parsley

### Instructions:

1. Preheat oven to 400°F. Place cod fillets in a baking dish and pat dry. Season with salt and pepper.
2. In a bowl, toss tomatoes with 2 tbsp olive oil, garlic, oregano, and salt and pepper. Arrange tomato mixture around the cod.
3. Drizzle remaining 2 tbsp olive oil over

the cod fillets.

4. Roast for 15-20 minutes until cod is opaque and flaky and tomatoes are bursting.
5. Remove from oven and garnish with chopped parsley before serving.

**Nutrition per Serving (1/4th recipe): Calories: 295 Fat: 16g Carbs: 4g Fiber: 1g Net Carbs: 3g Protein: 36g**

## Coconut Vegetable Curry

**Prep Time: 20 mins Cook Time: 25 mins Total Time: 45 mins Servings: 6**

**Ingredients**:

- 2 tbsp coconut oil
- 1 onion, diced
- 3 cloves garlic, minced
- 1 tbsp grated ginger
- 2 tbsp red curry paste
- 1 lb cauliflower florets
- 2 bell peppers, sliced
- 1 cup sliced mushrooms
- 1 can (13.5 oz) full-fat coconut milk
- 1/4 cup vegetable or chicken broth
- 1 tbsp fish sauce

- Juice of 1 lime
- Chopped cilantro for garnish

**Instructions**:

1. In a large pot or skillet, heat the coconut oil over medium heat. Sauté the onion for 2-3 minutes.
2. Add the garlic, ginger and red curry paste. Cook for 1 minute more.
3. Add in the cauliflower, bell peppers, mushrooms, coconut milk, broth and fish sauce. Bring to a simmer.
4. Reduce heat and simmer for 20-25 minutes, until veggies are tender but still crisp.
5. Remove from heat, stir in the lime juice and garnish with cilantro.
6. Serve over cauliflower rice if desired.

**Nutrition per Serving (1/6th recipe): Calories: 225 Fat: 19g Carbs: 10g Fiber: 4g Net Carbs: 6g Protein: 4g**

**Keto Chicken Enchilada Bake**

**Prep Time: 20 mins Cook Time: 30 mins Total Time: 50 mins Servings: 6**

**Ingredients**:

- 1.5 lbs boneless skinless chicken thighs, cooked and shredded
- 1 cup shredded cheddar cheese
- 1 cup shredded pepper jack cheese
- 10 oz enchilada sauce or salsa
- 1/2 tsp chili powder
- 1/2 tsp cumin
- 1/4 tsp garlic powder
- Salt and pepper to taste
- Chopped cilantro for topping

For the creamy sauce:

- 1 cup heavy cream
- 4 oz cream cheese, softened
- 1/4 tsp xanthan gum (optional)

**Instructions**:

1. Preheat oven to 375°F. In a bowl, mix together the shredded chicken, cheeses, enchilada sauce and spices.
2. Spread half the chicken mixture in a 9x13 baking dish.
3. In another bowl, whisk together the cream, cream cheese and xanthan gum until smooth. Pour half over chicken.
4. Top with remaining chicken mixture, then remaining creamy sauce.
5. Bake for 25-30 minutes until bubbling

around edges.

6. Remove from oven and let rest 5 minutes before serving. Top with cilantro.

**Nutrition per Serving (1/6th recipe): Calories: 495 Fat: 40g Carbs: 6g Fiber: 1g Net Carbs: 5g Protein: 34g**

## Macadamia-Crusted Mahi Mahi

**Prep Time: 15 mins Cook Time: 12 mins Total Time: 27 mins Servings: 4**

### Ingredients:

- 4 mahi mahi fillets (6 oz each)
- 1 cup macadamia nuts, finely chopped
- 1/2 cup almond flour
- 1 egg, beaten
- 1 tbsp olive oil
- Salt and pepper

For the Lemon Garlic Butter:

- 4 tbsp butter
- 2 cloves garlic, minced
- 2 tbsp lemon juice
- 2 tbsp chopped parsley

**Instructions**:

1. Pat the mahi mahi fillets dry and season both sides with salt and pepper.
2. Prepare two shallow dishes - one with the beaten egg and one with the macadamia nuts mixed with almond flour.
3. Dip each fillet first in the egg, then in the nut mixture, pressing gently to adhere.
4. In a skillet over medium-high heat, warm the olive oil. Cook the mahi mahi for 3-4 minutes per side until nuts are browned and fish is opaque throughout.
5. Transfer fillets to a plate and tent with foil. In the same skillet, make the butter sauce by melting the butter with garlic for 1 minute. Remove from heat and whisk in lemon juice and parsley.
6. Serve mahi mahi fillets with the garlic lemon butter sauce spooned over the top.

**Nutrition per Serving (1 fillet with 1/4 butter sauce): Calories: 520 Fat: 45g Carbs: 8g Fiber: 4g Net Carbs: 4g Protein: 29g**

## Keto Beef & Chorizo Stuffed Peppers

**Prep Time: 20 mins Cook Time: 40 mins**
**Total      Time:      1      hour**
**Servings: 6**

**Ingredients**:

- 6 bell peppers, halved lengthwise and seeds/membranes removed
- 1 lb ground beef
- 8 oz ground chorizo
- 1/2 cup riced cauliflower
- 1/2 cup shredded cheddar
- 1/2 cup shredded mozzarella
- 2 cloves garlic, minced
- 1 tsp chili powder
- 1 tsp cumin
- 1 tsp dried oregano
- Salt and pepper to taste

**Instructions**:

1. Preheat oven to 375°F.
2. In a skillet over medium-high heat, cook the ground beef, chorizo and garlic until browned and crumbled. Drain excess fat.
3. Transfer meat mixture to a bowl and mix with riced cauliflower, shredded cheeses, chili powder, cumin, oregano and season with salt and pepper.

4. Stuff each pepper half evenly with the meat mixture.
5. Place stuffed peppers in a baking dish and bake for 35-40 minutes until peppers are very tender.
6. Garnish with extra shredded cheese, chopped cilantro or sour cream if desired.

**Nutrition per Stuffed Pepper Half: Calories: 340 Fat: 22g Carbs: 7g Fiber: 2g Net Carbs: 5g Protein: 23g**

## Southwestern Shrimp Zucchini Boats

**Prep Time: 20 mins Cook Time: 15 mins Total Time: 35 mins Servings: 4**

## Ingredients:

- 4 medium zucchini, halved lengthwise
- 1 lb shrimp, peeled and deveined
- 1 cup cherry tomatoes, halved
- 1/2 cup chopped red onion
- 2 cloves garlic, minced
- 2 tsp taco seasoning
- 2 tbsp olive oil
- 1 avocado, diced
- 1/4 cup chopped cilantro

- 2 oz crumbled queso fresco or feta

**Instructions**:

1. Preheat oven to 400°F and scoop out seeds from zucchini to create boats. Brush with 1 tbsp olive oil and season with salt and pepper. Roast cut-side up for 15 mins.
2. Meanwhile, heat remaining 1 tbsp oil in a skillet. Saute the shrimp with taco seasoning for 2-3 minutes until opaque. Remove to a plate.
3. In the same skillet, saute the onions for 2 minutes then add the garlic for 1 min. Remove from heat and stir in tomatoes, cilantro and avocado.
4. Fill zucchini boats with shrimp then top with veggie mixture. Sprinkle with queso fresco.
5. Return to oven for 5 mins to heat through. Serve immediately.

**Nutrition per Serving (2 stuffed zucchini halves): Calories: 315 Fat: 17g Carbs: 16g Fiber: 6g Net Carbs: 10g Protein: 23g**

## Keto Beef Shawarma Bowls

**Prep Time: 25 mins Cook Time: 10 mins**
**Total Time: 35 mins Servings: 4**

**Ingredients**:

For the beef:

- 1 lb beef sirloin or ribeye, thinly sliced
- 2 tbsp olive oil
- 1 tsp cumin
- 1 tsp coriander
- 1/2 tsp cinnamon
- 1/2 tsp garlic powder
- 1/2 tsp salt
- 1/4 tsp black pepper
- 1/4 tsp cayenne

For the bowls:

- 4 cups riced cauliflower
- 1 cup diced tomatoes
- 1 cup diced cucumber
- 1/4 red onion, thinly sliced
- 1 avocado, diced
- 2 oz crumbled feta
- 2 tbsp chopped parsley
- Tahini dressing for serving

**Instructions**:

1. In a bowl, toss the sliced beef with

olive oil and shawarma spices until fully coated.

2. Heat a skillet or grill pan over high heat. Cook the seasoned beef in batches for 1-2 minutes per side until charred but still pink in the center.

3. To assemble bowls, divide the riced cauliflower between 4 bowls. Top each with sliced beef, tomatoes, cucumbers, red onion, avocado, crumbled feta and parsley.

4. Drizzle each bowl with 2-3 tbsp tahini dressing before serving.

**Nutrition per Serving (1 bowl): Calories: 415 Fat: 26g Carbs: 11g Fiber: 6g Net Carbs: 5g Protein: 33g**

## Keto Cabbage Lasagna

**Prep Time: 20 mins Cook Time: 1 hour Total Time: 1 hr 20 mins Servings: 8**

**Ingredients**:

- 1 large head green cabbage, leaves removed
- 1 lb ground Italian sausage
- 4 oz cream cheese, softened

- 1/2 cup grated parmesan
- 1 egg
- 1 tsp Italian seasoning
- 1 tsp garlic powder
- 1/2 tsp salt
- 1/4 tsp pepper
- 2 cups Rao's marinara or low-carb marinara
- 2 cups shredded mozzarella

**Instructions**:

1. Preheat oven to 375°F. Bring a large pot of salted water to a boil and blanch the cabbage leaves for 2-3 minutes until just tender. Drain and set aside.
2. In a skillet over medium-high heat, cook the sausage until browned and crumbled. Drain excess fat.
3. In a bowl, mix together the cooked sausage with cream cheese, egg, parmesan, Italian seasoning, garlic powder, salt and pepper.
4. Spread 1 cup of marinara sauce in the bottom of a 9x13 baking dish. Lay a layer of cabbage leaves overlapping to cover the bottom.
5. Top with half the meat mixture in an even layer. Spread 1 cup marinara over the top and sprinkle with 1 cup

mozzarella.
6. Repeat with another layer of cabbage, meat, marinara and cheese.
7. Cover with foil and bake for 40 minutes. Remove foil and bake 15 more minutes until melty.
8. Let rest 10 mins before slicing and serving.

**Nutrition per Serving (1/8th recipe): Calories: 420 Fat: 31g Carbs: 9g Fiber: 2g Net Carbs: 7g Protein: 24g**

# Soups

### Creamy Cauliflower Soup

**Prep Time: 15 minutes Cook Time: 30 minutes**
**Servings: 4**

**Ingredients**:

- 1 head cauliflower, cut into florets
- 4 cups chicken or vegetable broth
- 1 cup unsweetened almond milk
- 2 cloves garlic, minced
- 1 tsp turmeric
- 1/4 tsp cayenne pepper

- Salt and pepper to taste
- 2 tbsp olive oil or ghee
- Fresh parsley for garnish

## Instructions:

1. In a pot, bring the broth to a boil. Add the cauliflower and cook until tender, about 10-12 minutes.
2. Transfer half the cauliflower and cooking liquid to a blender. Add the almond milk, garlic, turmeric, cayenne, salt and pepper. Blend until smooth and creamy.
3. Return the pureed mixture to the pot with the remaining cauliflower pieces. Heat through.
4. Stir in the olive oil/ghee and adjust seasoning as needed.
5. Garnish with parsley before serving.

**Nutrition per serving: Calories 203, Fat 14g, Carbs 13g, Fiber 5g, Protein 7g**

## Spicy Thai Coconut Soup

**Prep Time: 10 minutes Cook Time: 20 minutes Servings: 4**

**Ingredients:**

- 2 cups chicken or vegetable broth
- 1 (13.5 oz) can coconut milk
- 1 inch fresh ginger, grated
- 2 cloves garlic, minced
- 1 lemongrass stalk, smashed
- 1 lb shrimp or chicken, diced
- 2 cups riced cauliflower
- 2 tbsp fresh lime juice
- 2 tbsp fish sauce
- 1 tbsp red curry paste
- 1/4 cup cilantro, chopped
- Salt and pepper to taste

**Instructions**:

1. In a pot, combine broth, coconut milk, ginger, garlic and lemongrass. Bring to a simmer.
2. Add the shrimp/chicken and cauliflower rice. Simmer until cooked through, 5-7 minutes.
3. Remove lemongrass stalk. Stir in lime juice, fish sauce, curry paste and cilantro.
4. Season with salt and pepper to taste before serving.

**Nutrition per serving: Calories 311, Fat 18g, Carbs 12g, Fiber 4g, Protein 25g**

### Roasted Butternut Squash Soup

**Prep Time: 15 mins Cook Time: 45 mins Servings: 4**

**Ingredients**:

- 1 large butternut squash, halved and seeded
- 2 tbsp olive oil
- 4 cups chicken or vegetable broth
- 1 cup unsweetened almond milk
- 1 tsp cinnamon
- 1/4 tsp nutmeg
- Salt and pepper to taste
- 2 tbsp pumpkin seeds for garnish

**Instructions**:

1. Preheat oven to 400°F. Rub squash flesh with 1 tbsp olive oil and season with salt and pepper. Place cut-side down on a baking sheet and roast for 40-45 minutes until very soft.
2. Scoop out squash flesh into a blender. Add broth, almond milk, cinnamon, nutmeg and remaining 1 tbsp olive oil. Blend until very smooth.
3. Transfer to a pot and heat through, adding more broth to reach desired consistency. Season with salt and

pepper.

4. Garnish with pumpkin seeds before serving.

**Nutrients Per Serving: Calories 194, Fat 10g, Carbs 21g, Fiber 5g, Protein 6g**

## Zuppa Toscana

**Prep Time: 10 mins Cook Time: 30 mins Servings: 6**

**Ingredients**:

- 1 lb Italian sausage, casing removed
- 6 cups chicken broth
- 1 bunch kale, stems removed and chopped
- 1 onion, diced
- 3 cloves garlic, minced
- 1/2 tsp red pepper flakes
- 1 cup cauliflower florets
- 1/2 cup heavy cream
- Salt and pepper to taste

**Instructions**:

1. In a large pot, brown the sausage over medium-high heat until cooked through, 5-7 minutes. Transfer to a

plate.

2. Drain off all but 1 tbsp fat from the pot. Add the onions and cook for 2 minutes until translucent.
3. Add the garlic and red pepper flakes and cook for 1 minute until fragrant.
4. Pour in the chicken broth and add the cauliflower florets. Simmer for 10 minutes.
5. Add the kale and cooked sausage. Simmer for 5 more minutes.
6. Remove from heat and stir in the heavy cream. Season with salt and pepper.

**Nutrients Per Serving: Calories 316, Fat 24g, Carbs 8g, Fiber 2g, Protein 17g**

## Beef and Vegetable Soup

**Prep Time: 20 mins Cook Time: 2 hours Servings: 6**

**Ingredients**:

- 1 lb stewing beef, cut into 1-inch cubes
- 8 cups beef broth
- 1 can (14.5 oz) diced tomatoes

- 1 onion, diced
- 3 carrots, sliced
- 3 stalks celery, sliced
- 2 cloves garlic, minced
- 1 tsp dried thyme
- 1 bay leaf
- Salt and pepper to taste
- 2 tbsp fresh parsley, chopped

**Instructions**:

1. In a large pot or dutch oven, brown the beef over high heat in 1 tbsp oil. Transfer to a plate.
2. Add a splash of broth to deglaze the pot, scraping up any browned bits.
3. Return beef to the pot with remaining broth, tomatoes, onions, carrots, celery, garlic, thyme and bay leaf. Season with salt and pepper.
4. Bring to a boil, then reduce heat and simmer for 1.5-2 hours until beef is very tender.
5. Remove bay leaf and stir in fresh parsley just before serving.

**Nutrients Per Serving: Calories 252, Fat 9g, Carbs 13g, Fiber 3g, Protein 28g**

## Creamy Garlic Mushroom Soup

**Prep Time: 10 mins Cook Time: 30 mins Servings: 4**

**Ingredients**:

- 1/4 cup butter or ghee
- 1 lb mushrooms, sliced
- 4 cloves garlic, minced
- 4 cups chicken or veggie broth
- 1 cup heavy cream
- 2 tbsp fresh parsley, chopped
- Salt and pepper to taste

**Instructions**:

1. In a large pot, melt the butter/ghee over medium-high heat. Add the mushrooms and garlic and sauté for 5-7 minutes until mushrooms are browned.
2. Pour in the broth and bring to a simmer. Cook for 15 minutes.
3. Remove from heat and use an immersion blender to puree the soup until desired smoothness.
4. Stir in the heavy cream and season to taste with salt, pepper and parsley.

**Nutrients Per Serving: Calories 314, Fat 28g,**

**Carbs 9g, Fiber 1g, Protein 8g**

### Broccoli Cheddar Soup

### Prep Time: 10 mins Cook Time: 30 mins Servings: 4

### Ingredients:

- 4 cups chicken or veggie broth
- 1 head broccoli, florets & stems chopped
- 1 small onion, diced
- 2 cloves garlic, minced
- 1/2 tsp dried thyme
- 2 cups shredded cheddar cheese
- 1 cup heavy cream
- Salt and pepper to taste

### Instructions:

1. In a large pot, bring the broth to a simmer over medium heat. Add the broccoli, onion, garlic and thyme. Cook for 10-12 minutes until broccoli is tender.
2. Use an immersion blender to puree the soup to your desired consistency (leave some broccoli chunks if you

prefer).

3. Whisk in the shredded cheddar and heavy cream until fully incorporated and melted.
4. Season with salt and pepper before serving.

Nutrients Per Serving: Calories 546, Fat 46g, Carbs 13g, Fiber 4g, Protein 23g

# Snacks and Desserts

**Avocado Chocolate Mousse**

**Prep Time: 10 mins Cook Time: 0 mins Servings: 4**

**Ingredients**:

- 2 ripe avocados
- 1/2 cup unsweetened cocoa powder
- 1/3 cup erythritol or monk fruit sweetener
- 1 tsp vanilla extract
- 1/4 tsp cinnamon
- 1/8 tsp sea salt
- 1/4 cup unsweetened almond milk (if needed)

**Instructions**:

1. Scoop avocado flesh into a food processor or blender.
2. Add cocoa powder, sweetener, vanilla, cinnamon and salt.
3. Blend until completely smooth, adding almond milk a tablespoon at a time if needed to thin out.
4. Portion into serving dishes and chill for 30 mins before serving.

Nutrition Per Serving: Calories 226, Fat 16g, Carbs 15g, Fiber 8g, Protein 4g

## Lemon Raspberry Fat Bombs

**Prep Time: 10 mins Cook Time: 0 mins Servings: 12 fat bombs**

**Ingredients**:

- 1 cup coconut butter
- 1/2 cup coconut oil, melted
- 1/4 cup fresh lemon juice
- 2 tbsp lemon zest
- 1/4 cup erythritol
- 1 cup fresh or frozen raspberries

**Instructions**:

1. In a bowl, whisk together the coconut butter, coconut oil, lemon juice, zest and erythritol until fully combined.
2. Gently fold in the raspberries.
3. Portion the mixture into silicon molds or a parchment-lined mini muffin tin.
4. Freeze for 30 mins until set. Store in the fridge.

**Nutrition Per Serving: Calories 130, Fat 13g, Carbs 3g, Fiber 1g, Protein 1g**

### Baked Curry Dill Cucumbers

**Prep Time: 10 mins Cook Time: 20 mins Servings: 4**

**Ingredients**:

- 4 cucumbers, cut into 1-inch slices
- 2 tbsp olive oil
- 2 tbsp fresh dill, chopped
- 1 tbsp curry powder
- Salt and pepper to taste

**Instructions**:

1. Preheat oven to 400°F.
2. Toss cucumbers with olive oil, dill, curry powder and salt/pepper on a

baking sheet.
3. Bake for 15-20 minutes until lightly browned and tender.
4. Serve warm or chilled.

**Nutrition Per Serving: Calories 93, Fat 6g, Carbs 9g, Fiber 2g, Protein 2g**

## No-Bake Coconut Lemon Balls

**Prep Time: 10 mins Cook Time: 0 mins Servings: 12 balls**

### Ingredients:

- 1 cup unsweetened shredded coconut
- 1/2 cup coconut butter, softened
- 2 tbsp lemon juice
- 2 tbsp lemon zest
- 2 tbsp erythritol
- 1/4 tsp salt

### Instructions:

1. In a bowl, mix together all the ingredients until fully combined.
2. Roll into 12 even balls and arrange on a parchment-lined plate.
3. Refrigerate for at least 30 mins before serving.

Nutrition Per Serving: Calories 106, Fat 10g, Carbs 3g, Fiber 2g, Protein 1g

## Keto Chocolate Chia Pudding

**Prep Time: 5 mins Cook Time: 0 mins (plus chilling) Servings: 2**

**Ingredients**:

- 1/4 cup chia seeds
- 1 cup unsweetened almond milk
- 2 tbsp cocoa powder
- 2 tbsp erythritol
- 1/2 tsp vanilla extract

**Instructions:**

1. In a bowl or jar, combine the chia seeds, almond milk, cocoa powder, erythritol and vanilla.
2. Mix very well, making sure there are no clumps.
3. Cover and refrigerate for at least 2 hours, stirring occasionally, until thickened to a pudding-like consistency.
4. Portion into dishes and enjoy chilled.

**Nutrition Per Serving: Calories 226, Fat 13g, Carbs 14g, Fiber 12g, Protein 7g**

## Keto Coconut Flour Pancakes

**Prep Time: 10 mins Cook Time: 15 mins Servings: 8 pancakes**

**Ingredients**:

- 1/2 cup coconut flour
- 1/2 tsp baking powder
- 1/4 tsp salt
- 4 large eggs
- 1/2 cup unsweetened almond milk
- 2 tbsp melted coconut oil or ghee
- 1 tsp vanilla extract
- 2 tbsp erythritol (optional)
- Butter or ghee for cooking

**Instructions**:

1. In a bowl, whisk together the coconut flour, baking powder and salt.
2. In another bowl, beat the eggs, then whisk in the almond milk, melted coconut oil/ghee, vanilla and erythritol (if using).
3. Pour the wet ingredients into the dry and mix until fully combined and

smooth.

4. Heat a skillet or griddle over medium heat and grease with butter or ghee.
5. Pour 1/4 cup portions of batter and cook for 2-3 minutes until bubbles form on the surface. Flip and cook 1-2 minutes more.

**Nutrition Per 2 Pancakes: Calories 220, Fat 16g, Carbs 10g, Fiber 6g, Protein 8g**

## Easy Keto Chaffle

**Prep Time: 3 mins Cook Time: 5 mins Servings: 1 chaffle**

### Ingredients:

- 1 egg
- 1/2 cup shredded cheddar cheese
- 1/2 tsp Italian seasoning or garlic powder (optional)

### Instructions:

1. Preheat a mini waffle iron or chaffle maker.
2. In a small bowl or ramekin, whisk together the egg and seasoning if using.

3. Fold in the shredded cheese.
4. Pour batter into the preheated waffle iron and cook for 4-5 minutes until golden brown.
5. Carefully remove chaffle and fill with your favorite keto fillings.

**Nutrition: Calories 321, Fat 25g, Carbs 2g, Fiber 0g, Protein 23g**


## Chocolate Keto Smoothie

**Prep Time: 5 mins Cook Time: 0 mins Servings: 1**

**Ingredients:**

- 1 cup unsweetened almond milk
- 2 tbsp almond butter
- 2 tbsp cocoa powder
- 1 scoop keto protein powder (optional)
- 1/4 tsp cinnamon
- 1 tbsp chia seeds
- 1 tbsp erythritol or monk fruit (optional)
- 1 cup ice cubes

**Instructions:**

1. Add all ingredients to a blender and

blend until completely smooth.
2. Taste and adjust sweetener if desired.
3. Pour into a glass and enjoy!

**Nutrition: Calories 406, Fat 34g, Carbs 15g, Fiber 10g, Protein 20g**

## Zucchini Nacho Chips

**Prep Time: 10 mins Cook Time: 15 mins Servings: 4**

**Ingredients**:

- 2 medium zucchinis, sliced 1/4" thick
- 2 tbsp olive oil
- 1 tsp chili powder
- 1/2 tsp cumin
- 1/2 tsp garlic powder
- 1/4 tsp cayenne pepper
- Salt and pepper to taste

**Instructions**:

1. Preheat oven to 425°F. Line 2 baking sheets with parchment.
2. In a bowl, toss the zucchini slices with oil and spices until fully coated.
3. Arrange in a single layer on the baking sheets.

4. Bake for 15-18 minutes, flipping halfway, until browned and crispy.
5. Let cool 5 minutes before serving. Serve with guacamole or salsa.

**Nutrition Per Serving: Calories 93, Fat 8g, Carbs 4g, Fiber 1g, Protein 1g**

## Blackberry Coconut Fat Bombs

**Prep Time: 10 mins Chill Time: 1 hr Servings: 12 fat bombs**

### Ingredients:

- 1 cup coconut butter, softened
- 1/2 cup coconut oil, melted
- 1/2 cup blackberries, mashed
- 1 tsp vanilla extract
- 1/4 cup erythritol
- 1/4 tsp salt

### Instructions:

1. In a bowl, mix together all ingredients until fully combined.
2. Scoop out mixture and roll into 12 even balls.
3. Place fat bombs on a parchment-lined plate and freeze for 1 hour to set.

4.  Once firm, transfer to an airtight container and store in the fridge for up to 2 weeks.

**Nutrition Per Serving: Calories 153, Fat 16g, Carbs 2g, Fiber 1g, Protein 1g**

# Dining Out Guide

While cooking at home allows you to fully control the ingredients, there are times when dining out is inevitable.

This section provides tips and strategies for navigating restaurants while sticking to your keto and anti-inflammatory nutrition principles.
Restaurant Tips

How to read menus and customize orders
Questions to ask servers about ingredients
Keto-friendly cuisines to look for
Beverages to choose or avoid

This section breaks down the best and worst options at different types of restaurants:

American/Steakhouse
Egg-based breakfasts, bunless burgers, steaks, green salads
Mexican
Fajitas with extra veg, salsa, guacamole; lettuce wrap tacos
Italian
Cheesy baked dishes like eggplant parm; zucchini noodles
Asian
Curry, pho, Vietnamese salad rolls, cauliflower rice stir-fries
Coffee Shops
Unsweetened coffees, teas, keto-friendly milk alternatives
Fast Food
Bunless burgers, salads with olive oil, hard boiled eggs

By arming you with specific menu hacks and low-carb, anti-inflammatory picks, you can be prepared when eating out. The section also covers decoding nutrition labels and managing workplace or social situations.

With the right strategies, you don't have to fall off track from your keto anti-inflammatory lifestyle when out of your normal routine. Planning ahead is key to making good choices.

# Stocking Your Keto Anti-Inflammatory Kitchen

To set yourself up for success on the keto anti-inflammatory diet long-term, it's crucial to have the right foods and tools on hand. This chapter covers:

## Pantry Essentials

Keto-friendly oils, vinegars, low-carb nuts, nut butters, spices
Fridge & Freezer
Fresh veggies, proteins, keto-friendly dairy, frozen seafood

## Tools & Gadgets

Chef's knives, avocado tools, veggie spiralizers, food processors
Meal Prep Tips
Batch cooking & freezing, component prep, food storage

## Shopping Lists

Comprehensive grocery lists for shopping efficiently

By stocking your kitchen with the right whole food ingredients and essential tools, you'll always be ready to whip up a nutritious keto anti-inflammatory meal.

The chapter also shares valuable make-ahead tips for batch cooking and freezing meals to streamline your routine. Having a well-stocked anti-inflammatory, keto-friendly kitchen makes this lifestyle a breeze.

With this comprehensive book covering every aspect of the keto anti-inflammatory approach - from the fundamentals and health benefits to an entire month's meal plan and a huge variety of recipes - you'll be fully equipped to transform your health while enjoying delicious, wholesome foods.

# Troubleshooting & FAQs

Making any major dietary change can come with its own set of challenges. This chapter aims to address common hurdles and questions that may arise when following a ketogenic, anti-inflammatory nutritional approach.

Troubleshooting Sections:

Keto Flu Remedies
Overcoming Carb Cravings
Dealing with Digestive Issues
Balancing Macros for Weight Loss Stalls
Combatting Fatigue & Brain Fog
Exercising on Keto
Managing Social Situations

FAQs Covered:

### Can I consume dairy on an anti-inflammatory diet?

While dairy can be inflammatory for some people, full-fat, unsweetened dairy like butter, ghee, and cheeses are generally allowed in moderation on a keto anti-inflammatory diet. However, those with sensitivities or allergies should avoid dairy completely. Dairy-free milk alternatives like unsweetened nut milks and coconut milk are good substitutes.

### How do I replenish electrolytes on keto?

It's important to replenish sodium, potassium, and magnesium when following a ketogenic diet. Salting foods liberally, consuming bone broth, and eating keto-friendly foods like avocados, greens, nuts, and seeds can help. Taking electrolyte supplements may also be beneficial, especially when first starting keto.

**What supplements are recommended?**

Some recommended supplements for a keto anti-inflammatory lifestyle include high-quality multivitamin, omega-3 fish oil, vitamin D3, magnesium glycinate, and exogenous ketones (esp when starting). Probiotic and digestive enzyme supplements can also be helpful. Always check with your doctor first.

**How much protein is too much protein?**

On a ketogenic diet, it's recommended to get around 0.6-1.0 grams of protein per pound of lean body mass. Going much higher than this can potentially cause issues like kicking you out of ketosis. Most people do well with 4-6 palm-sized portions of protein per day.

**How do I avoid keto flu symptoms?**

The "keto flu" of fatigue, headaches, brain

fog, etc when transitioning to keto can be minimized by staying hydrated, replenishing electrolytes, getting enough sleep, easing into carb restriction, and being patient as your body adapts to burning fat. Exogenous ketones may also provide relief.

## Why am I not losing weight on keto?

There can be several reasons for a weight loss stall, including not being in a calorie deficit, consuming too many nuts/nut butters, dairy sensitivity, snacking, and needing to recalculate macros. Be patient, analyze your food journal, and make adjustments as needed.

## How can I make keto more affordable?

Planning meals, buying in bulk, shopping sales, choosing affordable protein sources like ground meat and eggs, and prepping food in advance can all make following a keto diet more budget-friendly. Intermittent fasting can also reduce food costs.

## Can children follow a keto diet?

With proper guidance from a pediatrician, nutritionist, and careful planning/monitoring, children can safely follow a well-formulated ketogenic diet for certain medical conditions like epilepsy and metabolic disorders. Otherwise, keto is generally not recommended for most growing kids.

Whether you're experiencing the temporary discomforts of keto flu or frustrated by a weight loss plateau, this section troubleshoots the most common keto hurdles. It also directly addresses frequently asked questions around balancing macros, supplements, exercise and other topics.

The goal is to equip you with strategies to overcome any potential roadblocks, so you can sustain the keto anti-inflammatory lifestyle smoothly. With the right preparation and mindset, you can avoid or quickly overcome any bumps in the road.

# Moving Forward & Resources

The final part is designed to help you take the knowledge and habits you've built to continue thriving on the keto anti-inflammatory nutritional approach long-term.

## Lifestyle & Mindset

Adopting a ketogenic anti-inflammatory way of eating is just one part of an overall healthy lifestyle.

**Here are some additional tips to support your journey:**

Stay Hydrated - Drink plenty of water and herbal teas to support digestion, energy levels, and detoxification. Aim for at least half your body weight in ounces of water daily.

**Prioritize Sleep** - Poor sleep increases inflammation and throws hormone levels off balance. Strive for 7-9 hours per night by adopting good sleep hygiene habits.

**Manage Stress** - Chronic stress weakens the immune system and promotes inflammation. Practice relaxing activities like meditation, yoga, deep breathing, journaling, etc.

**Move Your Body** - Incorporate a variety of anti-inflammatory exercises like walking, light strength training, mobility work, and low-impact cardio. Avoid over-training.

**Connect with Others** - Having a strong support system is vital. Join online communities, meet up with like-minded friends, or find an accountability partner.

**Be Patient** - Healing takes time. Don't get discouraged. Trust the process and celebrate every non-scale victory like improved energy, better sleep, etc.

# Preferences

1. Longo, V. D. (2018). The longevity diet. Penguin.

2. Sisson, M. (2017). The keto reset diet. Harmony Books.
3. Moore, J., & Westman, E. C. (2014). Keto cure: The ketogenic diet and nutritional solution. Victory Belt Publishing.
4. Gundry, S. R. (2017). The plant paradox: The hidden dangers in "healthy" foods that cause disease and weight gain. Harper Wave.
5. Seaman, D. R. (2020). The Deflame Diet: Beating Inflammation for Better Health, Weight Loss, and Longevity. Rodale Books.

Journal Articles:

6. Forsythe, C. E., et al. (2008). Comparison of low fat and low carbohydrate diets on circulating fatty acid composition and de novo lipogenesis. Obesity, 16(11), 2456-2463.
7. Volek, J. S., et al. (2009). Carbohydrate restriction has a more favorable impact on the metabolic syndrome than a low fat diet. Lipids, 44(4), 297-309.
8. Schwingshackl, L., & Hoffmann, G. (2014). Long-term effects of low-fat

diets either low or high in protein on cardiovascular and metabolic risk factors: a systematic review and meta-analysis. Nutrition journal, 13(1), 1-15.

9. Venegas-Calerón, M., et al. (2021). Anti-inflammatory nutrition and inflammation: A review of current evidence. Clinical Nutrition, 10(4), 1057-1068.

10. Goldberg, E. L., & Dixit, V. D. (2015). Drivers of age-related inflammation and strategies for healthspan extension. Immunological reviews, 265(1), 63-74.

Printed in Great Britain
by Amazon

56570842R00066